What you really need to know about

HORMONE REPLACEMENT THERAPY

Dr. Robert Buckman

with Wendy Dear

Introduced by John Cleese

LEBHAR-FRIEDMAN BOOKS

New York • Chicago • Los Angeles • London • Paris • Tokyo

Lebhar-Friedman Books
425 Park Avenue
New York, NY 10022

A Marshall Edition
Conceived by Marshall Editions
The Orangery
161 New Bond Street
London W1Y 9PA

First U.S. edition published 2000 by Lebhar Friedman Books.
First published in the U.K. in 1999 by
Marshall Publishing Ltd.
Copyright © 1999 Marshall Editions Developments Ltd.

Library of Congress Cataloging-in-Publication Data

Buckman, Robert
    What you really need to know about hormone replacement therapy / Robert Buckman,
with Wendy Dear ; presented by John Cleese
    p. cm. -- (What you really need to know)
    Includes index
    ISBN 0-86730-798-6 (alk.paper)
    1. Menopause--Hormone therapy. I. Dear, Wendy. II. Title.

RG186.B79 2000
618.1'7506--dc21   99-043764

Originated in Italy by Articolor
Printed in and bound in Italy by New Interlitho

Project Editor: Alison Murdoch
Additional Editing: Jill Cropper
Indexer: Stephen Fall
Art Editor: Louise Morley
Picture Research: Carina Dvorak
Managing Editor: Anne Yelland
Managing Art Editor: Helen Spencer
Design Assistance: Joanna Dalby
Editorial Director: Ellen Dupont
Art Director: Dave Goodman
Editorial Coordinator: Ros Highstead
Production: Nikki Ingram, Anna Pauletti
DTP: Lesley Gilbert

Edited and designed by Phoebus Editions, 72-80 Leather Lane, London EC1N 7TR.

The consultant for this book was Shari Leipzig, M.D., who is an obstetrician and gynecologist
in general practice in New York City. She is also a clinical instructor of obstetrics and gynecology
at Mt. Sinai School of Medicine.

Contents

Foreword

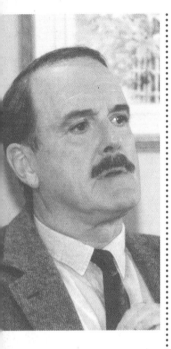

Most of you know me best as someone who makes people laugh.

But for 30 years I've also been involved with communicating information. And one particular area in which communication often breaks down is the doctor/patient relationship. We have all come across doctors who fail to communicate clearly, using complex medical terms when a simple explanation would do, and dismiss us with a "Come back in a month if you still feel unwell." Fortunately I met Dr. Robert Buckman.

Rob is one of North America's leading experts on cancer, but far more importantly he is a doctor who believes that hiding behind medical jargon is unhelpful and unprofessional. He wants his patients to understand what is wrong with them, and spends many hours with them—and their families and close friends—making sure they understand everything. Together we created a series of videos, with the jargon-free title *Videos for Patients*. Their success has prompted us to write books that explore medical conditions in the same clear, simple terms.

This book is one of a series that will tell you all you need to know about your condition. It assumes nothing. If you have a helpful, honest, communicative doctor, you will find here the extra information that he or she simply may not have time to tell you. If you are less fortunate, this book will help to give you a much clearer picture of your situation.

More importantly—and this was a major factor in the success of the videos—you can access the information here again and again. Turn back, read over, until you really know what your doctor's diagnosis means. In addition, because in the middle of a consultation you may not think of everything you would like to ask your doctor, you can also use the book to help you formulate the questions you would like to discuss with him or her.

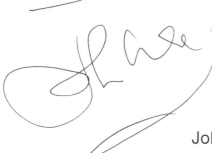

John Cleese

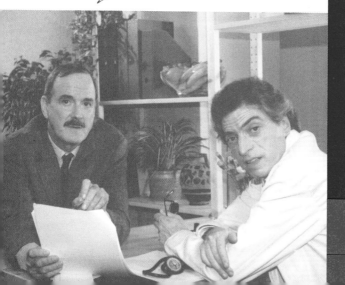

Introduction

DOs AND DON'Ts

Find out as much as you can about the subject so you can make an informed choice about HRT.

Don't be afraid to ask questions and seek help.

Hormone replacement therapy has a long history but for the last 20 years or so it has offered women the chance to make the change from one stage of life to the next much easier. Menopause is a fact of life for every woman born, yet each one may have a different experience at this time. One purpose of HRT is to help a woman manage the change well.

Menopause marks the end of a woman's child-bearing years and the beginning of a new chapter in her life. A woman who reaches the age of 50 today may live for another 30 years or more during which time her status and activities may alter considerably. Another purpose of HRT is to help a woman maintain good health in her later years.

Information and support

During the reproductive years, whether a woman has children or not, her health concerns tend to relate to the way her hormones function. These give her body vital protection though she may not be fully aware of it until menopause arrives and the symptoms of a lack of hormones are noticed. The prime female hormone, estrogen, is fascinating. As more and more research is done, its complicated, and highly important, role in the health of the body is revealed.

HRT is primarily a preventive health measure, used to protect the body against the disabling illnesses that can appear in later years. You will read more about each of them in the pages of this book.

So how do you decide about HRT? How do you balance the risks against the benefits? It must be an individual decision based on the best information you can get. The right doctors and nurse practitioners can help you decide how to make the choice by looking closely at your own situation. This book will arm you for such discussions. You will know more about what is happening to your body at this time and what may happen in the future if you have certain risk factors.

You will also have the information you need about the different types of HRT, how they work, and what you can expect from them. With HRT no decision need ever be final. The choice can be made at any age. With the information provided by this book you become a partner in your own treatment.

A normal life

Remaining as healthy as you can will be one of your prime concerns after menopause, for this ensures your independence as you get older. Whether or not to use HRT is one of the decisions you will need to make about your health and quality of life in the years ahead. It may be as important as good nutrition and exercise.

This is a time of new beginnings. You may become a grandmother, may take up opportunities to travel, study, or pursue other new challenges. The years after menopause should be yours to enjoy, in health.

NATIONAL OSTEOPOROSIS FOUNDATION

There are 275,000 new osteoporotic hip fractures each year in the United States. This organization publishes a range of pamphlets about osteoporosis and will provide contacts for local support groups. See page 78 for details of this and other useful organizations.

Chapter

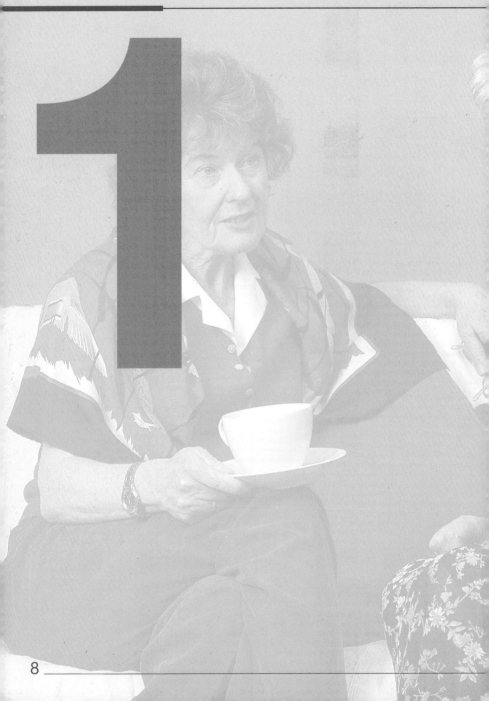

SYMPTOMS &
CAUSES

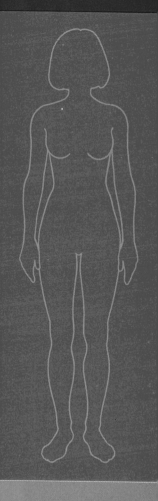

What is menopause?

Most women reach menopause a year before or after 51.

The World Health Organization defines menopause as the date of the final period, diagnosed retrospectively one year later.

In most women the whole process takes about four years.

The timing of menopause cannot be predicted—but some women will have experiences similar to their mother's.

Menopause occurs when a woman's ovaries produce no more eggs to be fertilized and the uterus stops its preparations for receiving them. It is one of her normal life processes and signals the end of the reproductive phase of her life that began at puberty.

What causes menopause?

Toward the end of a woman's reproductive years, her body starts to slow production of the two hormones vital to natural reproduction—estrogen and progesterone. As production of these hormones decreases, the ovaries gradually shrink until they are the grape-like size they were before puberty.

It is relatively rare for menopause to happen suddenly. It is more likely to be a gradual process during which menstruation is irregular and eventually ceases. The time span in which this occurs is called the climacteric (commonly called the change of life), and the perimenopause is the time closest to a woman's last menstrual period.

For over 95 percent of women the average age is 51. Women who smoke may begin the transition at an earlier age and their climacteric may be shorter.

What causes early menopause?

Very early menopause, before the age of 40, may occur as a result of medical or surgical treatment. This may be after having both ovaries removed, after a hysterectomy in which one or both ovaries are left in place but the uterus is removed, or after chemotherapy or radiotherapy has been used to treat a malignant disease.

Premature ovarian failure can sometimes happen spontaneously, and the cause is not always discovered.

HORMONES AND MENSTRUATION

HORMONE INTERACTION

In the first two weeks of a menstrual cycle, follicle-stimulating hormone (FSH) helps an egg cell (ovum or oocyte) in the ovary to mature. When the egg is ready to break out of its follicle, the amount of FSH reduces as luteinizing hormone (LH) takes over to complete the process called ovulation—when the egg is released.

By the time a woman reaches menopause, few eggs remain, and the hormone levels tend to fluctuate more wildly, which causes periods to be irregular.

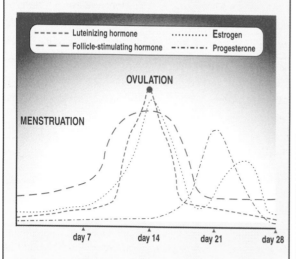

Between puberty and menopause the monthly cycle is affected by four related hormones whose levels all fluctuate during the cycle. The function of the gonadotrophins—FSH and LH—is to stimulate production of the other two hormones, estrogen and progesterone.

The effects of menopause

Menopause is not an illness but an important stage of a woman's life. However, the hormonal changes that take place at this time can have long-term effects on health in later life. Estrogen receptors have been found on nearly all tissues within the body and changing levels of estrogen have widespread effects. What this means to the body has yet to be fully studied but information is available on the bones and the circulation (see p. 42). Knowing what could happen to these vital parts will help you understand why hormone replacement therapy is considered a great advance in preventive medicine.

How are bones affected?

Osteoporosis is a condition in which the bones become porous and liable to fracture. Bones—like the rest of our bodies—consist of living tissue that breaks down and is constantly renewed. The two reproductive hormones—

THE EFFECTS OF OSTEOPOROSIS

There are half a million tiny sites in the body where bone is constantly being lost and remade. When age-related loss of bone occurs, bones can become weak and brittle. This loss of bone mass increases the risk of fracture, especially in the bones of the hips, wrist, and spine.

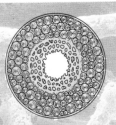

A healthy bone (above) has a strong outer layer of compact bone and plenty of soft, spongy bone rich in blood vessels in the center.

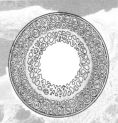

In an osteoporotic bone (above), the layer of compact bone becomes thinner and weaker and the spongy bone more porous.

estrogen and progesterone—are essential to this process of renewal. Other hormones—calcitonin and parathyroid hormone—also have their role to play.

From menopause onward, women lose bone density rapidly and there may be no symptoms until they suffer a fracture after a trivial injury. Progressive spine fractures lead to deformity, loss of height, and pain; hip fracture can be disabling and lead to loss of independence.

What gives bones their strength?

The strength of your bones is established in young adulthood through a combination of factors. These include a healthy lifestyle, a diet made up of a wide variety of foods and rich in calcium, daily exposure to sunlight (from which you obtain vitamin D), and regular weight-bearing exercise. All types of weight-bearing exercise, including brisk walking, have repetitive movements that place a strain on the skeleton and this in turn stimulates the bone-making process. The muscles also need to be strong to give the bones stability and help your balance, particularly in later life to prevent falls.

What can affect a bone's strength?

Before menopause several things can adversely influence a woman's bone mass (the bones' density and strength). The first is irregular, infrequent, or complete lack of periods (amenorrhea), which disturb the egg-releasing cycle (ovulation) and reduce the availability of estrogen and progesterone needed for bone. Period problems occur with polycystic ovary syndrome and illnesses such as anorexia nervosa or exercise-induced amenorrhea, as seen in gymnasts. Some treatments, such as for endometriosis, may cause amenorrhea.

The effects of menopause

The effects of menopause

Osteoporosis can be the result of either hormone deficiency or long use of steroids.

The gradual change in the bones is not painful until a fracture occurs; as a result osteoporosis is known as a "silent disease."

Can I minimize the risks?

If you are advised to have treatment that involves inducing amenorrhea you should ask the specialist to explain for how long your period will be stopped, the risks involved, in the short or long term, and what action can be taken to minimize the risks.

What else affects bone mass?

The eating disorders, anorexia nervosa and, to a lesser extent, bulimia, can also cause periods to stop. Over-enthusiastic aerobic exercising and athletics are another cause of amenorrhea, and this type of estrogen deficiency causes the bones to weaken prematurely. If a woman undertakes intensive physical workouts while not eating foods that contain calcium—such as milk, cheese, yogurt, sardines, and broccoli—the mineral content of her bones can be badly affected.

Smoking and drinking alcohol to excess are also known to damage bone-building cells and to bring on menopause about two years earlier than the average age of 51.

When are bones at their strongest?

Bones reach their peak mass between the ages of 20 and 30, the result of bone-making during childhood and adolescence. The level of your own bone mass will depend on several factors: the efficiency of the hormones involved, your state of health, your genes, and your lifestyle. Failure to reach the optimal peak bone mass is a major factor in osteoporosis. From about the age of 35 bones are subject to persistent mineral loss, a situation that is made worse by the lack of estrogen at menopause and after.

Are there any warning signs?

Unfortunately the gradual change in the bones tends not to be noticed until a fracture occurs. A short, thin post-menopausal Caucasian or Asian woman who has lost height, particularly between the waist and the shoulders, or is developing a hunch back, or kyphosis, has the classic signs of the disease. Osteoporosis is less common in African and Caribbean women.

There are two types of osteoporosis, one of which appears at an earlier age than the other, but both are treated in the same way (see pp. 30–31, 40–41).

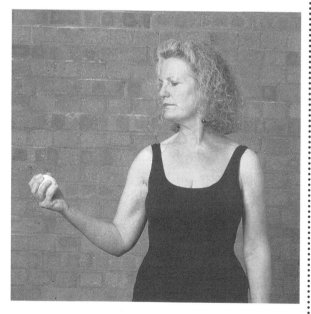

All forms of exercise will help to build stamina and improve balance, but weight-bearing types, such as brisk walking and the various types of racket sports, are most beneficial for bones. Squeezing a tennis ball for several minutes a day is a simple but useful exercise to do at home, to improve both your muscle strength and grip.

YOU REALLY NEED TO KNOW

◆ Even if your mother or another close relative suffered from osteoporosis, your chances of developing the disease may depend on other risk factors or lifestyle.

◆ The bones that thin and get weaker fastest are the long ones in the arms and legs and the small ones in the spine (vertebrae), all of which are more susceptible to fracture.

◆ In older people, fractures are usually the result of a fall, often caused by a loss of balance, tripping over an object, or confusion arising from taking prescribed drugs.

The effects of menopause

The effects of menopause

✓ HRT is one of the most important tools available to help women at menopause.

✓ It may be essential to long-term health to make lifestyle changes well before menopause.

It is rare for premenopausal women to fall prey to heart disease. Yet for women over 50, it is the single most common cause of death, just as it is for men. As life expectancy increases and people over the age of 50 make up a greater proportion of the population, medical attention is focusing more and more on this vulnerable area of the body.

Since the early days of hormone replacement therapy, its long-term use—five to ten years—has been promoted as providing protection against osteoporosis and cardiovascular disease (that is, disease of the heart, lungs, and blood circulation). The evidence to back its role in protecting bone mineral density has come from many studies and while there are alternatives to reduce fractures, HRT remains the favored treatment for the

ESTROGEN AND THE CARDIOVASCULAR SYSTEM

Until menopause, the hormone estrogen acts to protect a woman's body against the major diseases of the cardiovascular system: coronary heart disease and stroke.

The circulating blood carries oxygen from the lungs to all the cells of the body

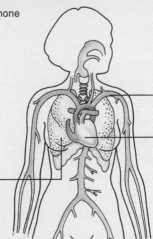

Estrogen prevents fatty plaques (atheromas) from sticking to artery walls, so blood flow to the brain and the rest of the body is not restricted

Estrogen keeps the muscular walls of blood vessels flexible, enabling the heart to pump blood efficiently

prevention of osteoporosis. To be fully effective, however, it is thought life-long use may be necessary. With heart disease and stroke the picture is not yet as clear, and research continues.

Estrogen and heart disease

It is known that during the reproductive years the estrogen circulating in a woman's body prevents fatty plaques (atheromas) developing within the artery walls. When less estrogen is produced, during menopause, these plaques, which are partly formed by excess cholesterol, start to develop and narrow the arteries so the heart has to work harder to push the blood through. Heart disease—coronary artery disease—occurs when the powerful heart muscle is disabled by the restricted blood flow.

Lack of estrogen is not the only factor involved in the development of atheromas. Your genes, general health, and lifestyle habits also contribute.

Estrogen and strokes

Strokes can happen at any age though it is most usually a condition of later years—that is, after menopause. A stroke occurs either because something blocks the blood flow to the brain or because there is bleeding in the brain. Atherosclerosis—narrowing of the blood vessels —in the brain, or in the neck leading to the brain, is the most common cause. The first sign of this may sometimes be "little strokes," transient ischemic attacks (TIAs), which last a few minutes and may be felt as numbness or tingling down one side of the body. The risk factors for stroke or TIAs are the same before and after menopause (see p. 42).

(see p. 42).

YOU REALLY NEED TO KNOW

◆ Angina is the most common symptom of heart disease in post-menopausal women.

◆ Exercising and giving up smoking are among the best things a woman can do for herself at menopause.

◆ As yet there is no clear-cut data about how effective HRT is in preventing either heart disease or stroke. But it is known that women using estrogen have better blood circulation and can exercise for longer.

The effects of menopause

The role of glands

✓ A woman's sexual development is controlled by the glands in the endocrine system.

✓ Hormones circulating in the blood affect both wellbeing and your general state of health.

✓ Menopause is triggered by hormonal changes in the endocrine system.

We all have two sets of glands—the exocrine and the endocrine. The exocrine system is made up of a number of glands connected directly to various organs by ducts. It is responsible for the production of tears, saliva, mucus, and sweat, as well as digestive juices from the pancreas and bile from the liver. In women it is involved in the production of milk (from the mammary glands), and in men the production of the fluid (from the prostate gland) that surrounds sperm in semen.

Glands and life-long health

The other system—the endocrine—is central to the way we grow, mature, and have children. In women these glands produce the female reproductive hormones, often called chemical messengers, which circulate in the bloodstream. They have a strong effect on your general day-to-day wellbeing and life-long state of health.

The pituitary gland, about the size of a pea, works with the hypothalamus, part of the brain, to organize the endocrine system. In conjunction with the thyroid, they control metabolism—the rate at which you burn calories to provide the energy your body needs to keep every cell in a state of good health through repair and maintenance.

The thyroid gland, which is in the neck in front of the windpipe, regulates the body's heating system. It also controls the way calories are used and the level of cholesterol in the blood.

Very importantly, through its hormone calcitonin, it co-ordinates the building of bones, working with the calcium and phosphorus regulators and parathyroid hormone produced by the four tiny parathyroid glands (located behind the thyroid). Correct levels of both minerals are needed in the blood for strong bones (see also p. 13).

A WOMAN'S ENDOCRINE SYSTEM

The different elements of the endocrine system have a profound effect on a woman's development.

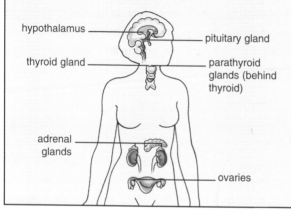

- hypothalamus
- pituitary gland
- thyroid gland
- parathyroid glands (behind thyroid)
- adrenal glands
- ovaries

How do hormones work?

The precise balancing act between the hormones is seen in the reproductive system, which, between puberty and menopause, provides at least one egg a month to be fertilized. At the time when the pituitary gland sets puberty in motion, two new hormones are produced. The hypothalamus stimulates the pituitary gland to send out follicle-stimulating hormone (FSH) to help an egg cell in the ovary to mature.

The follicle in which the egg grows releases estrogen to thicken the lining of the uterus, or endometrium. The pituitary then activates luteinizing hormone (LH) which bursts the follicle to release the egg into the fallopian tube. A cellular structure forms on the burst follicle and this produces progesterone, which prepares the uterus for the arrival of the fertilized egg.

Effects of hormone loss

✓ With falling estrogen levels, many parts of the body, including the skin, bones, and bladder, start to show changes.

✓ One definition of menopause is "the loss of ability to release a fertilizable egg."

In its role in the menstrual cycle, the female hormone estrogen keeps the walls of the vagina moist and in shape, ensuring that the skin in the area is thick and well lubricated. From puberty onward, estrogen gives a woman's body its curves, helps with the distribution of fat on the thighs and upper arms, and gives structure to the breasts. It also directly affects the walls of the arteries, preventing fatty plaques from forming and thus reducing the risk of coronary heart disease.

Does all the estrogen disappear?

The production of estrogen slows but does not stop completely at menopause. The amount that is produced depends on the amount of fat stored in your body. After menopause most of the body's estrogen comes from the fat cells, so a layer of fat is both protective and productive when the ovaries have ceased to function.

The quantity of estrogen produced is much less than during the reproductive years, and estrogen from fat cells is not as potent as ovarian estrogen, which was stimulated by the pituitary gland. The adrenal glands (on the kidneys) also produce some estrogen.

What happens to the progesterone?

If, after menopause, your body is not producing enough progesterone (which is only produced after ovulation and protects the lining of the uterus, or endometrium), you may experience the effects of having too much estrogen. An imbalance between the hormones estrogen and progesterone may cause what seem to be premenstrual syndrome (PMS) symptoms. It can also be the cause of sudden weight gain or bloating, similar to that which you may have experienced during your menstrual cycle. Fluid retention in the hands and around the stomach is not uncommon.

One school of thought considers that this imbalance of estrogen and progesterone occurs as a result of the action of xenoestrogens (estrogen-like substances absorbed through food that mimic the natural hormone). Phytoestrogens are plant hormones that also mimic estrogen (see p. 22). Naturopaths say that a diet with plenty of these can block the xenoestrogens.

(see p. 22)

HOW THE BODY IS AFFECTED

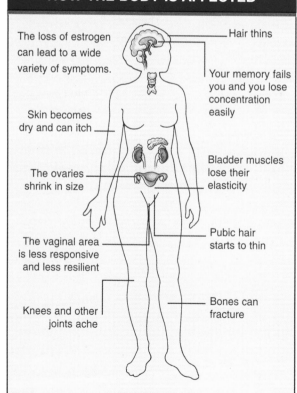

The loss of estrogen can lead to a wide variety of symptoms.

Hair thins

Your memory fails you and you lose concentration easily

Skin becomes dry and can itch

Bladder muscles lose their elasticity

The ovaries shrink in size

Pubic hair starts to thin

The vaginal area is less responsive and less resilient

Knees and other joints ache

Bones can fracture

YOU REALLY NEED TO KNOW

◆ Natural estrogen (estradiol), extracted from wild yam and soy, is also available in pill form.

◆ Estrogen is the most widely used prescription drug in the United States.

◆ Skin creams and implants are among formulations of estrogens and progestins (progestogens) used in Europe.

Effects of hormone loss

Symptoms of hormone loss

✓ Without estrogen, some body tissues, including those of the vagina, lose elasticity and shrink.

✓ Physiological changes after menopause can make sex less pleasurable.

Lack of hormones can cause various symptoms, although some women do not experience any of them.

Physical symptoms

Dry, itchy skin is a common complaint. You may feel as if your skin is "crawling" or it may become sweaty and hot. Some women find they react differently to being in the sun and get heat rash or hives. Some find the deodorant they've used for years suddenly stops being effective.

You may experience problems with your teeth, such as bleeding gums, loose teeth, or abscesses, and eyes may be dry and itchy. Your vagina may not lubricate naturally and be unresponsive, so that intercourse is painful. Even the thought of sex may worry you. You may have frequent urinary problems, such as cystitis, with

HORMONES AND YOUR DIET

Phytoestrogens are substances that are similar in their chemical make-up to natural estrogen. Two of them—known as lignans and isoflavones—are found in many plant foods including linseeds, whole-grain cereals, and bran, vegetables, fruits, soybeans, chickpeas, and other legumes.

These foods feature heavily in the Japanese diet and interest in them was aroused after studies conducted in Japan showed that menopausal women have a low incidence of adverse physical symptoms. Japanese women also suffer

less coronary heart disease and cancer of the breast, colon, and endometrium (lining of the uterus) than women in western countries, although this alters when they go to live in the West and abandon their traditional diet. This low incidence of menopausal symptoms and cancers may, of course, be due to other aspects of Japanese lifestyle or genetics, and more research is being undertaken, but there is evidence that a balanced diet, rich in phytoestrogens, can be beneficial to women at the time of menopause.

burning and itching, and you may experience "leaking" of urine when you laugh, sneeze, or run (this mostly affects mothers whose babies were delivered vaginally). Your internal temperature gauge may seem to go haywire so that you feel very hot one minute and cold and clammy the next. Night sweats are common.

Hair can become thin, limp or oily, and the scalp itchy or bumpy. Your facial hair, which has been almost invisible until now, may become apparent around the mouth or along the jawbone. Odd, longer hairs can suddenly sprout from pores on the chin.

You may find yourself putting on weight, around the waist as well as on the hips, thighs, and shoulders, and you may feel bloated and retain fluid, particularly in the week before you have or would have had your period. You may also feel unusual aches in your joints.

Emotional symptoms

You may find yourself more irritable than usual, or anxious about things that would not normally bother you. You may have difficulty making decisions and have feelings of unworthiness.

Your sleep pattern may go awry; you may suffer from insomnia or find yourself waking in the early hours filled with anxiety. You may feel depressed for no obvious reason and have difficulty getting your feelings back to normal or you may find it hard to concentrate.

Your memory may let you down and you may have to struggle to recall a person's name or a particular word or what you had gone upstairs to collect. You may suffer from unusual lack of confidence and mood swings, and you may feel unexpectedly tearful, yet your eyes may be dry and itchy at the same time.

1

YOU REALLY NEED TO KNOW

◆ Low levels of estrogen can cause an increase in sexual problems (e.g. vaginal dryness, pain, burning sensation).

◆ The ovaries also make testosterone, partly responsible for libido (sex drive). After a hysterectomy and post menopause the levels of this hormone drop.

◆ Emotional symptoms are not necessarily due to a lack of hormones. You should discuss any such symptoms further with your doctor or nurse practitioner.

Symptoms of hormone loss

Symptoms of hormone loss

Give up smoking: menopausal symptoms may appear several years earlier in women who smoke.

Keep a diary of symptoms to help you monitor the way your body is reacting at this time.

How will it affect me?

You may get some, many, or none of the symptoms that indicate the end of fertility. The physical and psychological effects may be severe and long lasting or irritating and short lived. In many cultures, the end of menstruation may be welcomed, because it allows women to take part in religious gatherings and prayers (from which they are barred while bleeding).

Menopause often coincides with major events in your life, such as children leaving home or relationship problems, and you may attribute your feelings to these events rather than to the changes taking place in your

WHAT A HOT FLASH REALLY FEELS LIKE

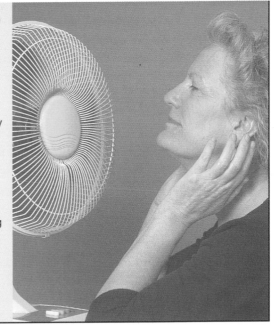

From the top of your scalp to the bottom of your feet you are suffused by heat then doused by a wave of sweat that feels surprisingly cold and makes your skin clammy. Several flashes may occur in a row, particularly at night, and you may become drenched in sweat. Daytime sweats, especially if they happen in company, can be embarrassing but the effects on you are not as noticeable as you think. Flashes are unpredictable and they can happen over several years.

body. Reassure yourself that you are healthy, that there is nothing unusual in what is happening to you, and that the symptoms can be alleviated.

What if I am on the pill?

The estrogens used in modern HRT are called "natural"—that is, they are the same estrogens (estradiol, estrone, and estriol) that the ovaries produce, but are artificially made or are obtained from other mammals. Women who take the combined oral contraceptive pill, which contains synthetic estrogens (chemically different and stronger than natural estrogens), may reach perimenopause or menopause without having any of the symptoms associated with constriction of the blood vessels (hot flashes, sweating) caused by changing hormone levels. This is because the amount of estrogen and progestogen in the contraceptive pill is greater than that of HRT. In the past, the pill was not prescribed to women over 35. Now, however, the modern low-dose type is regarded as safe for healthy non-smoking women who are not overweight and have no other risk factors.

How can HRT help?

The purpose of hormone replacement therapy is to keep your hormone levels steady long term and to protect against osteoporosis, heart disease, and stroke. Your body will function much as it did before the ovaries stopped producing estrogen and progesterone, and because these hormones are being replaced you should not experience the range of symptoms listed on pages 22–23. There is a wide range of HRT available; some types cause a regular bleed, others do not. Most doses have been found to protect bones against osteoporosis.

Symptoms of hormone loss

Chapter

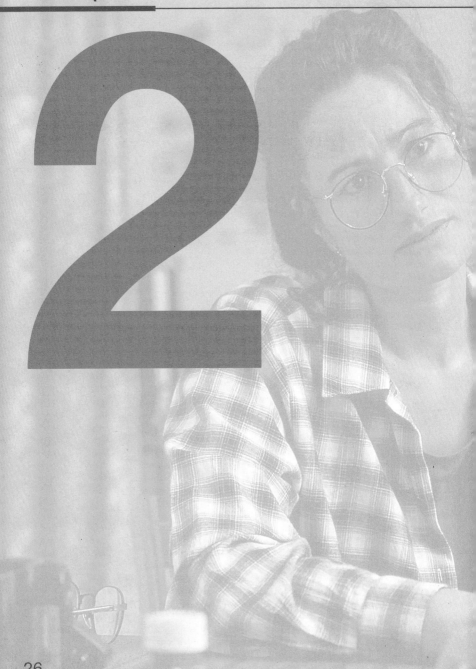

ASSESSMENT & DIAGNOSIS

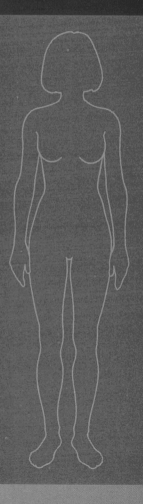

Tests a doctor might do

When you go to the doctor with your symptoms, a medical history will be taken and a physical examination done before any tests are ordered. It is best if you are not menstruating at the time of the appointment.

Pelvic examination

The doctor will want to assess your reproductive organs and estimate the size of your ovaries and uterus. Without hormonal influence, these shrink and after menopause will be the same size as they were before puberty. The examination takes little time and involves four actions: visual inspection and palpation (feeling) of the glands in the area; insertion of a speculum to hold the vaginal walls open so the cervix and vagina can be inspected (it is then removed); for the bimanual exam of the uterus the doctor uses a gloved hand for the vagina and presses down on the abdomen with the other hand; the other hand is then gloved to examine the rectum.

Cervical and breast tests

Women who are sexually active are advised to have a cervical smear test (Pap smear) annually, done when the speculum is in place during the pelvic examination. Breasts are examined by practitioners at the time of the Pap smear or more often if necessary. Mammography (breast X ray) should be done yearly after the age of 40; the radiologist may do a breast exam at the same time.

Blood tests

If your doctor needs more information, she may arrange for a sample of blood to be taken for analysis. A high level of follicle-stimulating hormone (FSH) in a woman under 40 could indicate premature ovarian failure; in a woman under 50 who has had a hysterectomy, the FSH level might usefully reveal the arrival of menopause. A woman over 45 with a uterus will not have blood hormone levels routinely tested because they fluctuate wildly at menopause and the results may not be of any help.

Blood tests may be done to screen for clotting risks (if there is a family history of thrombosis) and to check cholesterol level, and liver and thyroid function.

Ultrasound

If you have a history of period problems or fibroids, the doctor may arrange for an ultrasound to assess the condition of your uterus and its lining before further discussion about HRT.

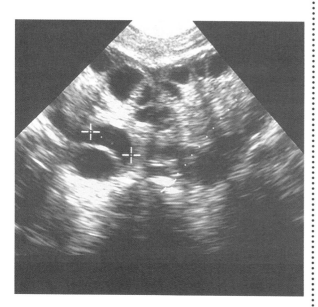

An ultrasound scan, like this one showing a uterus, uses sound waves to examine and take pictures of internal organs. It takes a few minutes to perform and does not use radiation.

YOU REALLY NEED TO KNOW

◆ Certain problems, which doctors describe as atrophic vaginitis, can badly affect your sex life at the time of menopause.

◆ The thinning of the skin in the area may make the vagina so sensitive that sexual intercourse is either very painful or not possible at all.

◆ A form of estrogen can be prescribed— as a cream or in the form of a silicone ring—to be used vaginally to relieve the symptoms of infections and vaginal discomfort.

Tests a doctor might do

Tests a doctor might do

FRACTURE FACTS

The wrist is the most common site for a fracture in pre-menopausal women. This fracture, called a Colles fracture, generally occurs when the woman puts her hand out to break a fall.

Older women are more likely to fall on and fracture their hip, which is disabling and can lead to a loss of independence.

If you have several risk factors for osteoporosis (see p. 40), your doctor may recommend that you have a bone density scan, often referred to as a DEXA (dual energy X ray absorptiometry).

How is a DEXA scan done?

The scanner uses very little radiation and the test is simple and quick to carry out. You don't need to get undressed for it, though you should wear loose-fitting clothes and remove your belt if you are wearing one. You lie on a bed with your feet raised (so the lower part of your spine is flat on the bed) while the X rays are taken

WHY A BONE DENSITY SCAN IS DONE

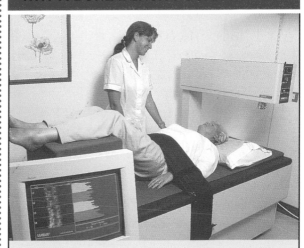

A bone density scan may be used to diagnose osteoporosis for the first time and then repeated a couple of years later to monitor progress after treatment has begun. It is a painless procedure that takes only a few minutes.

and the measurements are recorded on a computer. The computer printout, measuring the bone density of your lumbar or thoracic spine, femur (thigh bone), or wrist against that of a healthy young adult woman, will indicate whether osteoporosis is present, if there's a risk of fracture in the future or, when combined with the fact of a previous fracture, show that osteoporosis is already established.

There are other tests that may be used more widely in the future to measure bone density. Broadband ultrasound attenuation (BUA), which concentrates on the mass of bone at the heel, is inexpensive to carry out, and uses no radiation. Radiogrammetry (RA) can rapidly scan a bone, for example in the finger, and assess an individual's fracture risk.

What happens next?

The results of your test or tests will be sent to your doctor, who will explain them to you and tell you whether there is a need for any treatment. You may be prescribed HRT to protect against the development of osteoporosis, or other drug treatments if HRT is not suitable. If the tests show you have osteoporosis, the options to be considered are hormonal therapy or non-hormonal treatment.

Once treatment has started, you may have a follow-up bone density scan to assess whether the prescribed therapy is working as expected and whether your bone mass is increasing. Improvement of several percent increase of bone mass per year should be found.

Examining the bone mass in women with several risk factors is a reliable way of determining whether a woman has bone loss or bone thinning (osteopenia).

YOU REALLY NEED TO KNOW

◆ A loss of bone density in women can be detected after six months without periods.

◆ New data suggest that tooth loss may be an early sign of osteoporosis. After menopause, loss of teeth is common in osteoporosis sufferers.

◆ Other studies are being done to discover if women taking estrogen therapy retain teeth longer than women not on the therapy.

Tests a doctor might do

Tests a doctor might do

TEST FACTS

The most common device used to measure blood pressure is called a sphygmomanometer.

The procedure is painless but relax your arm and breathe evenly when the cuff is being put on.

Another important annual check, your blood pressure (BP) is measured as a matter of routine at menopause.

Blood pressure measurement

The nurse or doctor wraps a cuff around your arm, above the elbow. The cuff is in turn attached to a pressurized gauge. The nurse or doctor inflates the cuff to raise the pressure and stop the blood flowing. She then gradually releases the pressure while listening to your pulse through a stethoscope and watching the column of mercury on the gauge. Two measurements are recorded when each of two characteristic sounds is

WHY BLOOD PRESSURE IS MEASURED

Blood pressure, in both men and women, tends to increase with age. While temporarily elevated blood pressure is unlikely to be a problem, persistently high pressure increases the risk of a stroke, heart attack, and heart failure. As an increase in blood pressure may not have any symptoms and can easily go undetected, doctors usually measure the blood pressure of menopausal and postmenopausal women at least once a year.

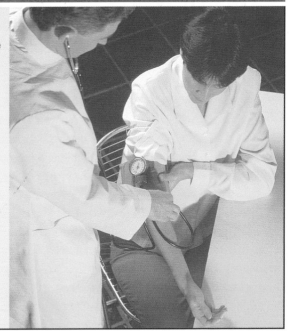

heard through the stethoscope. The first, higher, reading is the systolic pressure, when the heart muscle contracts, and the second, lower, reading is the diastolic pressure, when the heart muscle relaxes. Both are an indication of the forces on the artery walls as blood travels through the body. The blood pressure of an average adult is around 120/80 or less.

What does high BP mean?

Blood pressure rises for various reasons. Running for a bus, driving a car, feeling stressed, smoking, or drinking several cups of coffee can all affect it—as can anxiety at the prospect of having your blood pressure taken. It's best if you sit for five minutes and relax before the measurement is done.

As we age, our arteries become less elastic, and blood pressure may be high for this reason alone, but an elevated BP can also be an indication of heart or other problems. You may have high blood pressure without any symptoms, and if your reading is above 140/90—borderline hypertension—your doctor may suggest ways of lowering it.

What can be done to lower BP?

There are a number of self-help measures you will be advised to take. If you are overweight, you will be encouraged to change your eating habits to reduce your weight. You should also cut down salt intake and drink alcohol only in moderation (one and a half drinks maximum daily, see p. 75). Smokers will be advised to give it up as the habit increases the risk of high BP. A regular exercise program can also help to lower blood pressure. If none of these work, you may be prescribed medication.

2

YOU REALLY NEED TO KNOW

◆ Hypertension means your blood pressure reading is above "normal". Hypotension means it is below "normal."

◆ Low blood pressure is not usually considered a health issue and is rarely treated unless it accompanies blood loss or dehydration.

◆ High blood pressure is a risk factor for some common conditions in older age.

Tests a doctor might do

Chapter

3

CHOOSING & USING

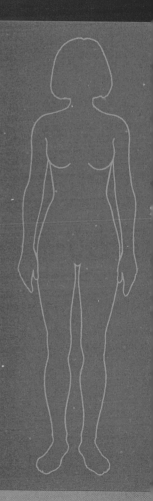

How do I find a doctor?

You have various options. Your neighborhood medical center may have a menopause or well-woman clinic, and you can always discuss the subject with the doctor or nurse there, who should be able to recommend the best course of action for you. If your medical center does not offer this service, the clinic time is inconvenient, or you do not wish to go through your doctor, try your local family planning clinic. Some run special menopause clinics where you can get information.

What should happen at your visit?

Ideally you will see a doctor or nurse practitioner, who will have allotted at least 30 minutes for the consultation, which will take place in private. She will take a detailed medical history, asking about previous pregnancies and contraception, if you have had a mammogram (breast X ray) recently and when you had your last cervical smear (Pap test).

She will also ask about the conditions you or members of your family have had, such as thrombosis, breast cancer, heart disease, fractures, thyroid, liver, bowel, or gallbladder problems. You will be asked whether you smoke, if you drink alcohol, and if so, how much per day, and about the type of exercise you do (if any).

You will be weighed, your height will be measured and your blood pressure taken. You will also have the opportunity to discuss any physical or emotional worries that you might have. Menopause often coincides with a time of personal turbulence and the doctor will want to be sure that the cause of your symptoms is ovarian failure with the resultant loss of hormones.

At this first visit you should ask as many questions as you want. It may be useful to write them down before you go to the doctor's office. You may be given brochures that will explain the various elements of menopause and treatment, and perhaps also a video.

What happens next?

At this point it may be sensible for you to leave and go home to read the brochures or watch the video. When you have had time to consider all the information and know which of it applies to your circumstances you can then make another appointment.

THE FIRST VISIT

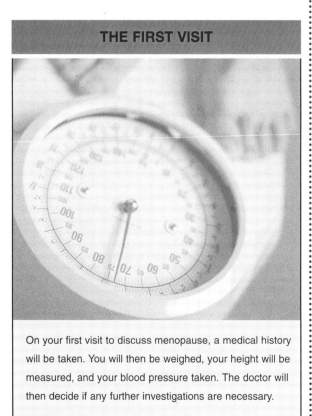

On your first visit to discuss menopause, a medical history will be taken. You will then be weighed, your height will be measured, and your blood pressure taken. The doctor will then decide if any further investigations are necessary.

YOU REALLY NEED TO KNOW

Questions you may want to ask your doctor include:

◆ How long will I have to wait for an appointment?

◆ How long do menopausal symptoms last?

◆ How will I know when I have passed menopause?

◆ What are the potential risks of using HRT?

◆ What side-effects should I expect?

◆ Will any side-effects gradually decrease?

How do I find a doctor?

How do I find a doctor?

DOs AND DON'Ts

✓ In the month before your appointment, record your symptoms, feelings, and problems.

✗ Don't be shy. If looking for a doctor ask friends for recommendations.

At the first or subsequent appointment you should have the opportunity to talk to the doctor about the treatment that would be considered most appropriate for you.

You may be asked further questions about the type of person you are and the kind of life you lead. This is important because it will help to establish the type of HRT that would be the most suitable for you.

Questions you may be asked at this point include: Are you good at remembering to take pills? Do you object to taking medication? Which symptoms worry you the most? Could you, if necessary, make lifestyle

YOU AND YOUR CLINICIAN

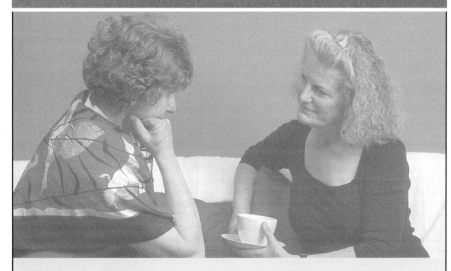

Menopause is an important issue because of the effect it can have on a woman's health for the rest of her life. Clinicians today should have time for you and understand how you feel. They should be willing and able to answer your questions, and offer up-to-date information freely for you to consider.

changes? Do you have realistic expectations of HRT and its purpose? Once the doctor has assessed your response to the questions she will tell you which type of HRT she thinks is most suitable for you.

If you decide you would like to start HRT, the doctor will talk you through the way it should be used and the signs you should watch for in the first few weeks. On the other hand, if you decide not to take up the option of HRT at this time you could discuss setting a date to review your decision in the future.

What if there are problems?

A good clinician will make sure you understand the purpose and importance of long-term, preventive treatment, and will encourage you to return at any time during the trial period (usually three months, but sometimes longer) if you are experiencing problems.

If you are having difficulties with the prescribed therapy, there is a wide-enough range available to choose another. This can continue if need be until you have settled with a therapy you are comfortable with— tailoring your therapy to your needs and lifestyle is the most effective way to ensure your long-term acceptance of the treatment.

Menopause is being taken more seriously today and women who are pre- or post-menopausal should be able to make an informed choice about the most suitable course of action for them. An understanding doctor will recognize that menopause can affect both you and your partner, and that you might want to bring your partner or a friend with you to discuss the options available to help you cope with the symptoms you are experiencing or protect your future health.

YOU REALLY NEED TO KNOW

Questions you may want to ask your doctor include:

◆ What type of problems might I experience?

◆ Will I still have a period each month?

◆ Can I call you to discuss the prescribed therapy if it doesn't suit me or should I make another appointment?

◆ How long should I stay on HRT?

How do I find a doctor?

Is HRT right for me?

Some types of gastro-intestinal surgery can prevent essential nutrients being absorbed, which can lead to bone problems.

Monitor your intake of milk and dairy products: women who do not get enough may lack calcium.

Women who are confined to bed through long-term illness are at greater risk of developing osteoporosis.

Your medical history

As you approach menopause, or even once you have reached it, it can help to take the time to weigh your possible risk of developing some of the conditions mentioned earlier. This will help you to make an informed decision, in conjunction with the professionals, as to whether HRT is right for you.

You know more about yourself and your family history than your doctor can ever know, but unless you have kept a detailed record of not only your own illnesses, but also those of close relatives, it may take some time to reveal it.

THE RISK FACTORS FOR OSTEOPOROSIS

Studies have shown that genetic, or inherited, factors account for approximately 70 percent of the risk of a woman developing osteoporosis in later life, but other factors will influence the outcome.

GENERAL FACTORS

◆ Early onset of menopause (before 45)
◆ A family history of the disease
◆ Prolonged absence of periods (six months or more) during the reproductive years (not including pregnancies)
◆ Long-term treatment with steroids (more than 7.5 mg/day for one year or more)
◆ Maternal history of hip fracture
◆ Asian or Caucasian background
◆ Long-term thyroid-replacement (e.g. for thyroid cancer)

As these details could have a bearing on your long-term health, it is worth spending some time collating all the relevant information before going to the doctor.

Will I develop osteoporosis?

One of the most debilitating of illnesses in later life is osteoporosis (see pp. 12-15). If there were symptoms of it or it was diagnosed in your own mother, sister, or father, HRT could be offered to you as a preventive therapy. Your own lifestyle will also have an effect. Check the risk factors listed in the box below.

The general and lifestyle indicators listed in this table also play a major part in determining whether or not a woman will develop the condition.

LIFESTYLE FACTORS

◆ Heavy smoking/drinking

◆ Lack of weight-bearing exercise

◆ Sedentary lifestyle

◆ Low intake of calcium

◆ Little exposure to daylight (vitamin D deficiency)

◆ Previous fracture (wrist, toe, ankle) after a minor injury

◆ Thyroid problems

◆ Digestive malfunction (i.e. chronic bowel disease, kidney or liver problems, or after gastrointestinal surgery)

◆ Prolonged periods of immobility due to chronic disease

YOU REALLY NEED TO KNOW

Your doctor will find the answers to the following questions about your mother's health history useful in making a diagnosis about your risk of developing osteoporosis:

◆ Did your mother grow smaller in old age?

◆ Did she ever fracture a bone?

◆ Did she develop a hunch back?

◆ Did she have an early menopause?

Is HRT right for me?

Is HRT right for me?

✓ Heart disease is the biggest cause of death in women over 45 in the United States.

✓ Using HRT reduces the risk of developing heart problems, but it is not yet clear by how much.

Your risks of heart disease

There have been a great number of studies, mostly in the U.S., on HRT and heart disease. But the results are not clear cut. In one, HRT users are 50 percent less likely to develop heart problems; in another it is 20 percent. The fact that over 300 risk factors have been identified puts the subject well beyond most people's understanding.

When you are considering whether HRT is right for you, there are two categories of common risks to look at: those you are born with, and those you can do something about. You can't change your genes, and if you have a family history of heart disease you may have inherited the tendency. The risk of developing heart disease increases with age, and in women this risk accelerates after menopause. Those who have had a very early menopause, before or just after 40, are especially vulnerable.

RISK FACTORS FOR HEART DISEASE

Your doctor can advise on reducing the risk of heart disease. Simple measures such as losing weight or stopping smoking can help, or you may need drug treatment for a medical condition such as high blood pressure (hypertension).

GENERAL FACTORS
◆ Family history of heart disease
◆ Age
◆ Premature menopause
◆ High blood pressure
◆ High cholesterol
◆ Being overweight
◆ Diabetes

LIFESTYLE FACTORS
◆ Smoker
◆ Sedentary occupation
◆ Little or no exercise
◆ Diet high in saturated fat
◆ Excess alcohol
◆ Stress

Next, look at your general health. The conditions that put you at risk of heart disease and stroke are: high blood pressure, high blood cholesterol, being overweight, and diabetes. Finally, list the aspects of your lifestyle that may cause damage. Do you smoke, do little or no exercise, eat lots of fatty foods, drink too much alcohol? Are you often stressed, do you have a sedentary job?

Making changes

Talk to your doctor about how to reduce your known risks. Giving up smoking, cutting down your alcohol intake, adopting a low-fat, low-salt diet, losing weight, and getting regular exercise will be the first recommendations.

Before menopause, your artery walls have the protection of estrogen, which also influences the level of blood fats (lipids, one of which is cholesterol). If you have an inherited cholesterol problem (called familial hypercholesterolemia), changing your diet to remove animal fats and eating more whole cereal grains, vegetables, and fruit may prevent an excess of the fat building up on the artery walls. Drug treatment can be prescribed if diet alone fails. One study showed that drug treatment used in conjunction with HRT had better results than either treatment used separately.

If you have diabetes mellitus—another high-risk factor for heart disease—and can get it under control with a high-fiber, low-fat, low-sugar diet or by taking pills or insulin, you can consider HRT. If you are overweight and can lose some of it, all the better.

The role stress plays in heart disease is not completely understood. As the years around menopause have their own physical and personal stress, finding ways to reduce its effect will always be in your best interest.

YOU REALLY NEED TO KNOW

◆ Illnesses that affected your mother, father, or near relatives may have an influence on your own health.

◆ There are only a few medical problems that might preclude you from taking HRT.

◆ If your condition can be treated and HRT would not be counterproductive, your doctor might prescribe it.

Is HRT right for me?

Is HRT right for me?

✓ The incidence of breast cancer increases as women age.

✓ All breast lumps should be checked by a doctor, but most are found to be non-cancerous.

Your risks of breast problems

Many women have "lumpy" breasts during their reproductive years, others suffer tenderness or pain. If any of these seem worse around menopause you should discuss the situation with your doctor. Lumps should always be checked out, although most turn out to be benign (not cancerous).

Breast cancer is both age- and estrogen-related. In particular, the less time a woman is exposed to her own reproductive hormones (from puberty to menopause), the lower her risk (see the box below left).

If you have, or have had, ovarian or digestive problems, your doctor will take these into account, but they are much less likely to rule out the use of HRT.

Your risk of ovarian problems

Ovarian conditions often do not have any obvious symptoms and may not be discovered until a woman

---

THE RISKS OF DEVELOPING BREAST CANCER

The risk of developing breast cancer in women taking long-term HRT is less than that reported from drinking two drinks of alcohol a day, smoking cigarettes, or being obese after menopause. Studies show that:

- after five years on HRT, there are 2 extra cancer cases per 1,000 women
- after 10 years on HRT, there are 6 extra cancer cases per 1,000 women
- after 15 years on HRT, there are 12 extra cancer cases per 1,000 women

While this demonstrates an increased incidence, there is no evidence that there are more breast cancer deaths.
Also the small increase in risk reduces after stopping HRT.

goes to her doctor with an apparent bowel or bladder problem. Cysts may be the cause.

If there is any hint of malignancy, a hysterectomy with removal of the ovaries will usually be advised. After a hysterectomy, it may be recommended that the woman consider using HRT.

Ovarian cancer rarely has symptoms until the tumor is advanced. As with breast cancer, if it occurs pre-menopausally there is a chance it may be inherited. The risk increases postmenopausally.

Your risks of thrombosis

If you or a close family member have a history of thrombosis (venous thromboembolism or deep vein thrombosis/DVT) you will need to weigh the risks against the benefits of using HRT. You can ask your doctor if a blood test of clotting proteins would be helpful in assessing your risk.

If you have no family history of thrombosis but if you are overweight or have extensive varicose veins, HRT may not be advised. DVT is relatively rare and the risk increases with age.

Digestive illnesses

Gastrointestinal surgery, or any condition treated with steroids, may have affected your bones, and this could influence the type of HRT offered. If a woman is genetically predisposed to colon cancer, her doctor may arrange for her to be screened. There is encouraging research on the bowel-protective role of HRT. Sigmoidoscopy is recommended for women every three to five years after 50 and colonoscopy for people with a family history of polyps or colon cancer.

YOU REALLY NEED TO KNOW

◆ Studies have revealed three cases of thrombosis per 10,000 users of HRT a year. The risk for non-users is one in 10,000.

◆ The risk appears to be greatest in the first year of oral therapy.

◆ Long-haul flying (more than four hours) increases the risk of DVT. HRT users might be advised to take half a tablet of aspirin just before the flight.

Is HRT right for me?

What about my weight?

HRT prevents weight gain around the waist and abdomen after menopause.

After menopause the lean body mass decreases and the fat mass increases.

Your weight at menopause is very important. Some "padding" on the body—on the hips, thighs, and shoulders rather than around the waist (see p. 64)—protects the bones of the skeleton and is a storage place for vitamin D, without which calcium cannot be absorbed and used by the bones. Cells in this layer of fat also produce a weak form of estrogen. However, this does not mean you should be overweight—you should try and keep your body weight as close to the ideal as possible.

How do I find my ideal weight?

Your doctor will weigh and measure your height, then use tables to work out your body mass index (BMI)—the

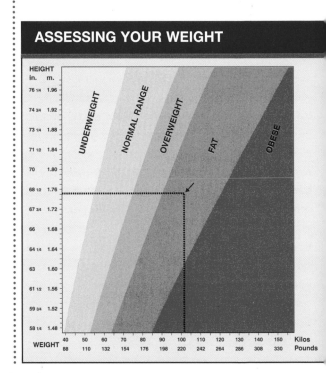

ASSESSING YOUR WEIGHT

ideal weight range for your height. Some fat is needed to protect the bones from osteoporosis, so a woman with a light frame and no excess fat during and after menopause, with a BMI below the normal range, may be at risk of developing the disease.

If you are at risk, a bone density scan may be done, and if the condition is diagnosed, treatment can be started. Treatment aims to reduce bone loss and the risk of fracture, with possible bone mass increase. HRT is effective in meeting all of these. If you have established osteoporosis, bone preservation is a priority. If you don't want HRT or it is contraindicated in your particular case, ask your doctor about other options (see p. 68).

You can use the chart on the left to work out your ideal weight for your height, and to see whether you are within the normal range or if you are under- or overweight. Find your height on the vertical axis and your weight on the horizontal. Where the lines meet gives you an instant assessment of whether you are a healthy weight. In the diagram, the lines meeting in the area designated as "fat" apply to someone 69 inches tall who weighs 220 lbs.

YOUR BODY MASS INDEX

Doctors may use the body mass index (BMI)—a ratio of your actual weight to your height. It is calculated by dividing your weight (in kilos) by your height (in meters) squared. A BMI of between 20 and 25 is healthy.

YOU REALLY NEED TO KNOW

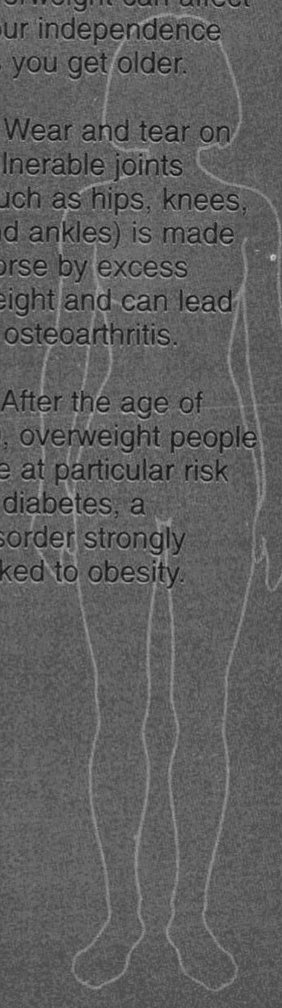

◆ The problems caused by being overweight can affect your independence as you get older.

◆ Wear and tear on vulnerable joints (such as hips, knees, and ankles) is made worse by excess weight and can lead to osteoarthritis.

◆ After the age of 50, overweight people are at particular risk of diabetes, a disorder strongly linked to obesity.

What about my weight?

When should I start HRT?

If you start HRT at least a year after menopause, therapy may be prescribed that will maintain your period.

Young women who have menopausal symptoms after a hysterectomy should be counseled about HRT.

If you decide to use HRT, the only answer to the above question can be "when you are ready," and this should not be before you have been given all the information you need about hormone replacement therapy.

Menopause is a normal event, a marker for the end of the reproductive years. However, a woman who reaches 50 today has every chance of living for another 30 or more years, and the quality of those years may be influenced by the changes that occurred in her body at or before menopause. When you talk to a nurse practitioner or doctor about your health now and in the future, both with and without HRT, be as frank as you can, and discuss your feelings and any anxieties.

WHO SHOULD NOT USE HRT?

If you have any of the conditions listed in the left-hand column it may mean that you should not use HRT:

- breast cancer
- cancer of the endometrium (lining of the uterus)
- abnormal vaginal bleeding of unknown origin
- liver disease
- ovarian cancer
- deep vein thrombosis
- pulmonary embolism
- otosclerosis
- pregnancy

If you have any of the conditions in the right-hand column, specialist advice may be needed:

- family history of thrombosis
- gall stones
- fibroids
- endometriosis (a condition in which fragments of the womb lining develop outside the uterus)
- osteoporosis (caused by the use of steroids)
- breast problems
- migraines
- epilepsy

You are much more likely to continue to benefit from the therapy if you have confidence in it, have made your own informed choice to use it, and know that you have the back-up of people who are interested in your well-being. It also helps to know that if one type of HRT is not suitable for you, you can try a different type.

How long should I use HRT for?

You can continue the therapy for the rest of your life, provided you see a doctor for regular check-ups. When properly administered, HRT is free of major side-effects and will continue to provide protection against osteoporosis and problems related to low estrogen.

Will I need to change my therapy?

The range of HRT available is constantly expanding, and your needs may change over time. It may be that the type of therapy that you were prescribed at, say, perimenopause is not the best at a later age. Making at least annual visits to your doctor who keeps up to date with all the new formulations, is the best way of finding out if you need to change.

If you were prescribed HRT at menopause and stopped using it after a short time, you may decide to start afresh later. Much will depend on whether there have been any major changes in your health during this time. See your doctor for advice on what is best for you. Whatever you do, don't just "give it a try" and then give up. Try it for three months and seek further medical advice if you are not happy. Often the problem is related to unrealistic expectations of the therapy. It is not a panacea for all ills, but aims to replace the hormones no longer produced by the ovaries.

3

◆ Making the decision to start using HRT should be based on knowledge of your own health and what can affect it.

◆ If you have realistic expectations of HRT you are more likely to continue to use it and to reap the long-term benefits.

◆ A woman who has had a premature menopause as the result of treatment for an illness needs to know if she should consider HRT.

When should I start HRT?

Types of HRT

Various forms of hormone replacement therapy meet different needs. In a perimenopausal woman who has a uterus, two hormones are used so that the uterus is kept healthy by mimicking the hormone output of the reproductive years. The difference is that with HRT, the shedding of the womb lining as a monthly bleed generally occurs at a regular, predictable time. Or it may not occur at all.

THE DIFFERENT FORMS OF HRT

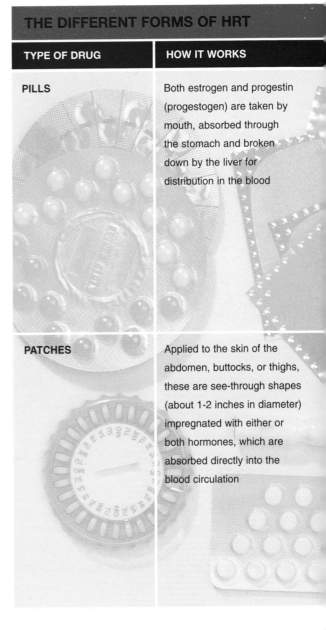

TYPE OF DRUG	HOW IT WORKS
PILLS	Both estrogen and progestin (progestogen) are taken by mouth, absorbed through the stomach and broken down by the liver for distribution in the blood
PATCHES	Applied to the skin of the abdomen, buttocks, or thighs, these are see-through shapes (about 1-2 inches in diameter) impregnated with either or both hormones, which are absorbed directly into the blood circulation

ADVANTAGES	DISADVANTAGES
• Simple to take	• May cause nausea and breast soreness
	• Hormone levels are not always constant
	• Requires a good memory as lapses negate intended effect
	• Must not be taken by women with liver disease
• Hormones don't need to be metabolized by the liver	• Can be annoying to apply
• Various strengths are available	• Need to be replaced at regular intervals
• Hormone levels are generally constant	• Obvious sign of therapy
	• Do not always stick well on thin, dry skin
	• May cause allergic reaction

YOU REALLY NEED TO KNOW

The group you are in indicates which type of HRT will suit you:

◆ A. Perimenopausal with a uterus
◆ B. Have had a hysterectomy (ovaries removed)
◆ C. Have had a hysterectomy (ovaries not removed)
◆ D. Postmenopausal with a uterus
◆ E. Postmenopausal without a uterus

◆ Group A: estrogen and progestin; will usually have periods.

◆ Groups B, C and E: estrogen-only therapy, without periods.

◆ Group D: continuous/combined estrogen/progestin therapy but will not always be free of periods.

Types of HRT

Types of HRT

The estrogens used in hormone replacement therapy—estradiol, estriol, and conjugated equine estrogens—are classed as natural (unlike the contraceptive pill in which synthetic hormones are used). The hormone progesterone is replaced by progestin (progestogen), a group of drugs similar to the natural hormone. If you have had a hysterectomy, you will probably receive only continuous estrogen.

THE DIFFERENT FORMS OF HRT

TYPE OF DRUG	HOW IT WORKS
INTRAUTERINE DEVICE (IUD)	A system (Progestasert) that releases progestin (levonorgestrel) to protect the uterus and simultaneously provides contraception for the perimenopausal woman
VAGINAL THERAPY (ESTROGEN CREAM)	Direct help for vaginal and urinary symptoms

ADVANTAGES	DISADVANTAGES

• Lasts for one year
• Convenient
	• Has to be fitted by a
	  doctor
	• Not licensed for HRT
	• Side-effects are irregular
	  bleeding or heavy periods
	  or cramps

• Choice of methods:
  cream or silicone ring
  (which is replaced every
  three months)
	• Not licensed for the
	  prevention of osteoporosis
	• Progestins may also
	  be needed in long-term
	  treatment

YOU REALLY NEED TO KNOW

◆ Local applications of estrogen are used to counter problems caused by aging (recurring urinary tract infections, vaginitis, and non-lubricating tissues, which prevent or make sexual contact difficult or painful).

◆ Conjugated estrogens come from the urine of pregnant mares and are more potent than lab-made estrogens.

◆ Progestins are synthetic versions of the female hormone progesterone.

HRT in pill form

Hormone replacement therapy in pill form is simple to take, but it is essential to follow the advice that is given with the packs, in particular when to take the pill and what to do if you miss a day. All oral therapy is licensed for the prevention of osteoporosis.

AVAILABLE RANGE OF PILLS

TYPE OF DRUG	BRAND NAMES
ESTROGENS	ESTRACE 306 and 721
	ESTRATAB 2421
	MENEST 2379
	OGEN 2567
	ORTHO-EST 1793
	PREMARIN
PROGESTINS	AMEN 839
	AYGESTIN 988
	CYCRIN 989
	PROVERA
	PROMETRIUM
ORAL ESTROGEN AND PROGESTIN	PREMPRO 2.5 mg
	PREMPRO 5.0 mg

Note: Brand names may vary.

GENERIC NAMES

micronized estradiol

esterified estrogens (principally estrone)

esterified estrogens (principally estrone)

estropipate

estropipate

conjugated estrogens and testosterone

medroxyprogesterone acetate

norethisterone acetate

medroxyprogesterone acetate

medroxyprogesterone acetate

medroxyprogesterone acetate

medroxyprogesterone

medroxyprogesterone

YOU REALLY NEED TO KNOW

◆ Estrogen and progestin tablets are packaged like the contraceptive pill with days of the week clearly shown so you know if you have missed taking one.

◆ If progestin is taken separately (with non-oral estrogen), the first day of the month is a good starting date as it is easy to remember the set number of days to take it.

◆ Oral therapy, being taken by mouth, is processed by the liver before entering the bloodstream.

HRT in pill form

HRT in patch form

Described as a transdermal system, patches contain estrogen (and sometimes progestin), which is absorbed through the skin into the bloodstream. The hormone strength in patches is too low to act as a contraceptive.

PUTTING ON A PATCH

1. Patches are individually wrapped. Tear the protective wrapper along one edge to remove oval or circular patch. Bend it so one half of the plastic backing can be pulled off.

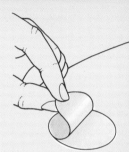

2. Without touching the sticky side, press the patch onto dry, hairless skin on the buttocks and pull off the remaining half of the backing.
Hold the patch in place for a short while to ensure it sticks.

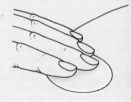

AVAILABLE RANGE OF PATCHES

TYPE	ESTROGEN AND PROGESTIN COMBINED
BRAND/ GENERIC NAMES	COMBIPATCH estradiol, norethindrone acetate Note: Brand names may vary.

WHERE TO APPLY

A patch should be placed on the thighs or buttocks, though not on the same area of skin twice in a row. Choose the least conspicuous area but ensure that it won't be covered by elasticated fabric, such as on the waist or underwear line, where friction might loosen it.

Your patch should not be affected by bathing, showering, swimming, or exercising, but may leave a mark on your skin from the adhesive, in the same way that a bandaid does. If you get a reaction to the adhesive, discuss this with your doctor.

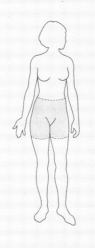

YOU REALLY NEED TO KNOW

◆ Patches are supplied in monthly packs marked with suggested change dates. The twice-a-week ones will say, for example, Mon/Thurs, Tues/Fri, and so on. You choose the days to start on. The once-a-week type will have the seven days displayed.

◆ If you are still having periods, the instructions will tell you on which day of your cycle to apply the patch.

◆ Mark the package in some way to remind you to change the patch on the same day or days.

ESTROGEN TRANSDERMAL SYSTEM (change twice a week)	ESTROGEN TRANSDERMAL SYSTEM (change once a week)
ALORA	FEMPATCH
ESTRADERM	CLIMARA
VIVELLA	

HRT in patch form

Other types of therapy

After the menopause specific therapy may be used to relieve symptoms. SERMs (selective estrogen receptor modulators) are an option when taking estrogen is contraindicated.

LOCALLY APPLIED HRT

TYPE	BRAND/GENERIC NAMES	
VAGINAL **CREAMS** Not generally considered to be complete hormonal therapy.	ESTRACE	estradiol
	OGEN 2570	estradiol
	PREMARIN	conjugated estrogens
	CRINONE 4% or 8%	progesterone (not approved for HRT)

Note: Brand names may vary.

ESTROGEN OR A SERM?

EFFECTS ON	HOT FLASHES	VAGINAL DRYNESS	BREAST	UTERUS
ESTROGEN	Reduces	Alleviates	Stimulates tissue growth, can cause breast tenderness	Stimulates tissue growth unless taken with progestin
RALOXIFENE	Doesn't help, may aggravate	No evidence that it alleviates	Does not stimulate breast tissue	Does not stimulate tissue growth

LOCALLY APPLIED HRT

Vaginal creams are not quite an alternative to systemic systems (for example pills or patches) and are mostly prescribed to relieve menopausal symptoms that adversely affect the vagina. Application varies depending on the condition. As some of the estrogen is absorbed into the bloodstream, with frequent use progestin may also be prescribed. Intravaginal estrogen is placed close to the cervix, using an applicator supplied with the cream.

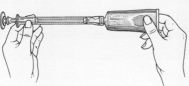

CARDIOVASCULAR SYSTEM	BONES
Boosts HDL (good) cholesterol, lowers LDL (bad). Appears to reduce heart disease risk	Increases bone density, helps reverse osteoporosis
Lowers LDL (bad) cholesterol. May increase risk of blood clots	Increases bone density (but less effectively than estrogen), helps prevent osteoporosis

**YOU REALLY
NEED TO KNOW**

◆ Period-free HRT, called "continuous combined HRT," was developed for women who still have a uterus and are post-menopausal. It provides therapy without "periods."

◆ In the first twelve months of new treatment, light spotting or bleeding may still occur.

◆ If the bleeding continues, there may be doubt about the date of your menopause. You may be advised to change to a sequential combined HRT (estrogen followed by progestin) for a while.

◆ If you continue to have irregular bleeding, you may need follow-up tests to evaluate this.

Other types of therapy

Chapter

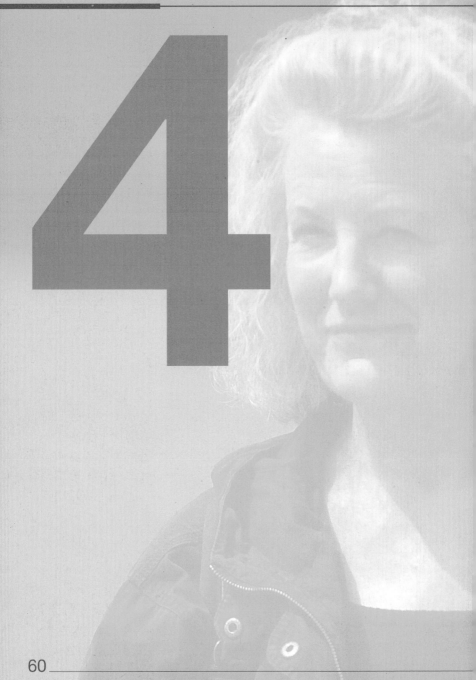

4

LIVING WITH HRT

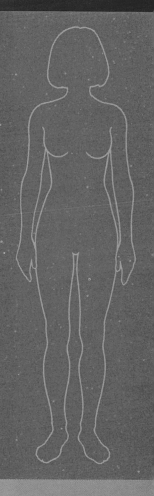

Your body and HRT

✓ While some symptoms of a lack of estrogen appear at menopause, others may not show until years later.

✓ Studies have shown HRT users have reduced incidence of age-related macular degeneration—the most common cause of blindness in older people.

Estrogen and the heart

Before menopause it is rare for a woman to have a high level of cholesterol in her blood (unless it is inherited, see p. 42). The female hormones circulating in the blood keep the levels of "good" cholesterol (HDL) up and "bad" cholesterol (LDL) down. Progesterone also controls the level of triglycerides (another type of fat), so the risk of atheromas forming is reduced.

Women who, before and at menopause, have no sign of coronary heart disease may benefit from the estrogen in HRT, possibly reducing their risk of developing it by up to a third. It is not so certain that secondary prevention (in women who have heart attacks after menopause) helps. If you are in this category, you can discuss your options with your doctor.

Estrogen and the bladder

Urinary incontinence and urinary tract infection are both common problems at, and after, menopause. These are uncomfortable, and often embarrassing, conditions that need medical attention.

Both result from lack of estrogen (see p. 20), which causes the lining walls of the bladder and urethra (the tube through which urine passes out of the body) to become thinner, drier, and vulnerable to infection. The tissues around the bladder neck also weaken, and this, combined with loss of muscle tone (a natural part of the aging process), results in stress incontinence (leaking a little urine when you laugh, cough, or run) or urge incontinence (the sudden feeling of needing to pass urine immediately). HRT may not improve incontinence in all cases; Kegel (pelvic floor) exercises may help (see p. 72) and surgery may be considered (see p. 73).

HRT and the cervix

The cells of the cervix change throughout a woman's life, under the influence of the reproductive hormones, but these changes slow at menopause when the body's production of estrogen and progesterone alters. However, smear tests are essential for women who have been sexually active. The earlier any change in cervical cells is detected, the more effective the treatment will be.

Cervical abnormalities are important at and after menopause, when cancer is most common. Hormones affect the cervix (making it more moist) and the ease of taking a smear, but not the abnormalities that can be detected.

THE HEART, CERVIX, AND BLADDER

Lack of female hormones has a crucial effect on some of a woman's vital organs.

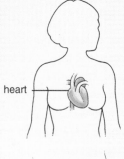

HEART
Without hormones to protect the artery walls, fatty deposits (atheromas) can build up

CERVIX
The area around the cervix shrinks through loss of support tissue

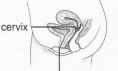

heart

cervix

BLADDER
You are more likely to leak urine when you laugh, cough, or run

└─ bladder opening

YOU REALLY NEED TO KNOW

◆ During what is known as "menstrual chaos"—when periods become erratic leading up to menopause—bleeding can be heavier or lighter than expected, and the cycles can be shorter or longer. Your doctor will want to rule out any abnormality (e.g. a polyp) before offering solutions.

◆ If you are perimenopausal, you may want to note physical and emotional symptoms for three months before attending a well-woman exam to find out what can be done.

Your body and HRT

Your body and HRT

When a woman is perimenopausal, fat on the hips and thighs is dependent on estrogen.

At menopause this fat is redistributed to the abdomen, which could explain why many women feel as if they are gaining weight at this time.

Gallbladder problems

Women are four times as likely as men to have gallbladder problems and they often appear during the 40s. The gallbladder collects bile produced by the liver to help with the digestion of fats. Among other things, bile contains cholesterol, and if there is too much of it, it combines with mineral salts to form gallstones.

When gallstones are tiny and sludge-like they may cause burping, a bloated feeling, and nausea after a meal. If they become large and pass into the bile duct leading from the gallbladder, they may become stuck. If this happens, severe pain, fever, and vomiting may result. If a woman has gallstones or gallbladder problems, HRT is usually not advised until the problems have been treated.

Although blood cholesterol levels before menopause are kept in check by the female reproductive hormones (as is fat distribution on the body), it is thought that there

YOUR SHAPE AT MENOPAUSE

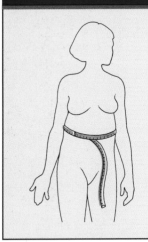

Some weight gain is common at menopause. However, excess weight around the stomach and waist—commonly called an "apple shape"—means that you are at greater risk of heart disease and gallbladder problems.

You can calculate your waist-to-hip ratio by measuring your waist at its narrowest point and your hips at their widest point. Divide your waist measurement by your hip measurement to get your waist-to-hip ratio. If your waist-to-hip ratio is above 0.8, it is worth trying to lose some weight.

is more cholesterol in the bile of overweight women. If you put on weight in your 40s it could increase your risk for gallbladder problems at and after menopause.

Effects of excess weight

If the fat you put on builds up around your abdomen rather than your hips and thighs, you may also be at risk of debilitating illnesses of older age

The results of a study of 13,000 adults aged between 29 and 59, conducted by the University of Glasgow, showed that anyone with a large waist size was four times more likely than average to develop late-onset diabetes and three times more likely to have heart disease. For women, the danger level is a waist over 35 inches (89 cm).

Estrogen and the mind

Like the breasts, blood vessels, and other organs, the brain has estrogen receptors and these may play a role in memory. The central nervous system, which is responsible for the senses of touch, sight, taste, smell, and hearing, sends messages from the skin, eyes, mouth, nose, and ears to the brain via nerve cells called neurons. There are gaps (called synapses) between the neurons, and chemical messengers (hormones) bridge these gaps to ensure the message gets through uninterrupted.

Lack of communication between neurons is a feature of memory loss and conditions such as dementia and Alzheimer's disease. Various trials have shown that postmenopausal women who are using HRT don't suffer as much memory loss as those not taking extra estrogen. And among women with Alzheimer's disease, the age of onset was later in those who had had some previous estrogen therapy.

YOU REALLY NEED TO KNOW

◆ Several studies have shown that while women tend to increase their body weight around the time of menopause, taking HRT does not lead to extra weight gain.

◆ Bloating and fluid retention are problems common to PMS and menopause. The cause is thought to be related to progesterone.

◆ If a woman is using HRT, she may blame this for weight gain instead of finding out if there could be other reasons for it.

Your body and HRT

Side-effects of HRT

SELF-HELP

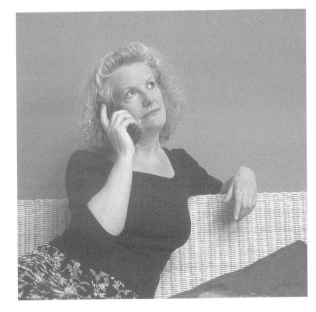

✓ Before you begin HRT you should have had the chance to talk to the doctor or nurse practitioner about possible side-effects.

✓ Being aware of what to expect will prevent unnecessary anxiety and will encourage you to persevere with HRT, rather than stopping before you have given the therapy a chance.

When you first start HRT, side-effects are quite common. The reason is usually the sudden rise in estrogen levels. For example, your breasts may feel tender, or you may have cramps in your legs, nausea, or headaches. If symptoms persist, talk to your doctor.

PMS symptoms

If you still have your uterus, you will be prescribed progestin, which is given with estrogen to protect the uterus lining. You may retain fluid and feel bloated, and you will have a period. This may not be the same as past bleeds, but you should be warned that it will happen.

You might find the side-effects unacceptable, but don't just stop taking the progestin—this can adversely affect the lining of the uterus. Go back to your doctor and discuss the situation.

If you are dissatisfied with your prescribed therapy, make an appointment with your doctor to discuss the problems so that a solution can be found.

Bleeding

When you first start using continuous combined therapy, which is intended to protect the uterus while eliminating periods, withdrawal bleeding can be a problem (and may require the use of tampons, pads, or panty liners). Bleeding can happen at unpredictable times and can be both irritating and inconvenient. This type of therapy is usually given for a three-month trial, so you should record the days of bleeding in your diary and report them at the follow-up appointment. If there is still bleeding after six to twelve months, action will be required.

The right therapy

If the chosen therapy is right for you, all your menopausal symptoms should disappear or be much less intense within days. After a few months of HRT you should have established a routine that feels natural and you should feel better. If this is not the case, go back to the doctor to discuss the reasons for this and to talk about the other options that may be more suitable.

Women's Health Initiative

One of the most important areas of investigation in the Women's Health Initiative is HRT and who would most benefit from it, and under what conditions. The U.S. government-sponsored study of women, all volunteers aged between 50 and 79, extends over fifteen years (it will be completed by 2007) and it aims to find ways to prevent three of the major causes of death and disability in postmenopausal women: heart disease, cancers, and osteoporotic fractures. The study should also help to resolve some of the questions related to the risks and benefits of long-term use of HRT.

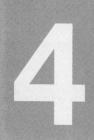

YOU REALLY NEED TO KNOW

◆ The range of HRT is wide and new types appear often. When you have a follow-up appointment you may wish to ask about them.

◆ On the horizon (not FDA approved yet in the U.S.) is tibolone, a synthetic combination of oral estrogen, progestin, and testosterone (to improve libido). For postmenopausal women, it is taken continuously and does not stimulate the womb lining so there is no monthly bleed. It prevents loss of bone density.

◆ Irregular bleeding can occur when changing from one type of HRT to another type.

Side-effects of HRT

Treatment for osteoporosis

Hormone replacement therapy is licensed to provide long-term protection against osteoporosis, a crippling condition that gets worse with age. Healthy women in their 60s and 70s may be well past menopause but can still use HRT or derivatives to protect their bones. If there are contraindications to HRT, other drugs and treatments (such as SERMs, see opposite) can be used.

DRUGS USED TO TREAT OSTEOPOROSIS

TYPE OF DRUG	PROS AND CONS
BISPHOSPHONATES (BRAND DIDRONEL, GENERIC ETIDRONATE; BRAND FOSAMAX, GENERIC ALENDRONATE)	These are mostly used to treat older women who have established osteoporosis and must have long-term treatment. Etidronate is for women with low bone density, with corticosteroid-induced and with established osteoporosis. Alendronate promotes new bone formation in established osteoporosis. To minimize side-effects of alendronate, the medication is taken on waking, with plain water, at least 30 minutes before any further food or drink.
CALCIUM AND VITAMIN D SUPPLEMENTS	On their own, calcium and vitamin D supplements are not considered to be effective in increasing bone mass, though they can help to prevent age-related bone loss. The supplements have to be taken together so that calcium can be absorbed by the body. The effect is better when the supplements are taken in conjunction with weight-bearing exercise.

Note: Brand names may vary.

TYPE OF DRUG	PROS AND CONS
CALCITRIOL	Useful in treating corticosteroid-induced osteoporosis, which occurs during long-term oral treatment for chronic illnesses such as asthma and arthritis. Rapid loss of bone density is a risk factor for people who take steroids for such illnesses. Calcitriol is taken as an inhalation.
CALCITONIN	Given as an injection into the muscles. It is helpful in relieving pain, a feature of severe osteoporosis following fracture of the spine, as well as preventing further bone loss, though it is not as successful as HRT or the bisphosphonate, alendronate, at increasing bone density.
SERMs (SELECTIVE ESTROGEN RECEPTOR MODULATORS) RALOXIFENE (EVISTA) TAMOXIFEN (NOLVADEX)	For postmenopausal women with osteoporosis and women with low bone density. SERMs mimic the action of estrogen on certain tissues of the body. They are not advised for women with current or a history of deep vein thrombosis and pulmonary embolism. See also p. 58.

YOU REALLY NEED TO KNOW

◆ SERMs are for older women, whose bones indicate risk of osteoporosis, but who cannot, will not, or should not use HRT, usually because of breast cancer risk.

◆ A SERM disables estrogen receptors in the breast and uterus (which means it doesn't affect them) while working with those in bone.

◆ The SERM raloxifene (Evista) stops bone loss and may promote bone repair. Taken in tablet form, it has some side-effects in the first few months, usually mild leg cramps and hot flushes. It does not treat symptoms of menopause.

Treatment for osteoporosis

Regular check-ups

X For over 90 percent of women who develop breast cancer the cause is unknown.

X It is estimated that between 5 and 10 percent of cancers are hereditary, but it is not known, even with gene testing, whether those women at risk will develop the disease.

The breasts of younger women are "denser," that is they have more fibrous or glandular tissue, than those of older women. Between the ages of 30 and 40, the composition of the breasts changes and they develop more fatty tissue, which starts appearing amid the glandular tissue. By the time of menopause, most of the glandular tissue—part of the reproductive process—has gone. If a woman is using HRT, her breasts remain similar to those of a woman in her 40s as a result of the prescribed hormones.

It is common practice for women's breasts to be checked by mammography every year from the age of 40. A premenopausal woman who is considering HRT should have a mammogram arranged by her doctor.

The purpose of these X rays is to look for changes in the breast and to follow up on anything unusual that may be seen. A woman going for screening will be asked if she is using HRT or if she has breast implants because both of these will help the radiologist who reads the X ray to understand more about the image that appears on the mammogram.

The importance of early detection

Of breast lumps found, only one in ten will be cancerous and most will not spread from the original site. Early detection and prompt treatment have the greatest effect on this type of breast cancer. It is also thought that breast cancers found in HRT users are less aggressive and the outcome is better than in those who develop breast cancer when not on HRT. It is a fact that breast cancer is a common illness of postmenopausal women, but the greatest risk of death for them is heart disease. While one in twenty-five women in the U.S. may die from breast cancer, one in two will die from heart disease.

Follow-up

Once you are settled on your type of HRT, your doctor should encourage you to be checked regularly, at least once a year. Prescriptions are not repeated automatically and a doctor's appointment will be needed for renewal. Your weight and blood pressure will be monitored, you will be advised on breast examination, and you will be asked about any side-effects you might be experiencing.

You will also have a pelvic examination. You should discuss any unusual bleeding. You may be asked about your lifestyle (how much regular exercise you get, for example) and if you have not yet gone through menopause, the subject of contraception may be discussed and the date of your next smear test checked.

HAVING A MAMMOGRAM

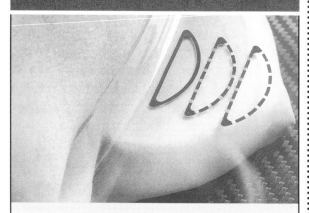

The X rays used in a mammogram penetrate only a few inches into the breast, and carry very little risk. Your breasts are compressed between two plastic plates during the procedure (shown above), which can cause mild discomfort.

YOU REALLY NEED TO KNOW

◆ Studies around the world are showing that HRT offers long-term protection against osteoporosis.

◆ HRT protects against endometrial, ovarian, and colon cancers.

◆ HRT is thought to improve gum health and thus reduce tooth loss.

◆ HRT may improve balance and help to maintain memory.

Controlling incontinence

Don't suffer in silence: incontinence can be helped by exercises, drugs, or surgery.

Incontinence gets worse at menopause because estrogen loss affects the muscles.

Some women suffer from urinary incontinence for many years without seeking help, because they are too embarrassed to discuss it. Yet it is exceedingly common, and you should appreciate doctors do understand the problem and the feelings it engenders.

There are two main types. Stress incontinence is the condition in which a small amount of urine leaks out when you are exercising or when you laugh, cough, or sneeze. With the other type, urge incontinence, you just can't hold back the need to pass urine by concentrating on something else or crossing your legs. Both may be related to loss of estrogen or can be the long-term result of giving

KEGEL EXERCISES TO TIGHTEN PELVIC FLOOR MUSCLES

These exercises improve the tone of the pelvic floor muscles and prevent "leaking" of small amounts of urine. Do them as often as you can every day—you can do them standing (while waiting for the train, for example) or sitting down (at your desk or when watching TV). If you have difficulties remembering to do them, write a note and stick it to the door of the refrigerator to remind you to do them while you cook dinner, or make a sandwich.

◆ Keep your legs slightly apart and close your back passage (anus) as if you were trying to avoid passing gas.

◆ At the same time, draw the front passage (vagina) inward and upward as if trying to stop passing urine. (Do this for real in the bathroom if you have problems with it.)

◆ Hold for a count to five, saying to yourself "a thousand and one, a thousand and two…" up to five.

◆ Relax for a count of five, then repeat ten times.

Once you can do this easily, increase the length of time you hold the passages closed. Your aim is to hold them closed for fifteen seconds.

birth vaginally. Incontinence can affect not just your social life but your sex life as well. The return of estrogen to the body through HRT may restore control in many women, but others may need more help to overcome the problem.

The doctor or nurse-practitioner at your clinic will explain the various methods that can be used. Ways of training the bladder may be suggested or medical intervention (e.g. drugs) may be advised. Doing pelvic floor exercises will be encouraged.

Is surgery necessary?

In some cases of incontinence you may be referred to a gynecologist, who specializes in urogynecology. In the past, surgery has been considered the best option to tighten the neck of the bladder, but another, less invasive, treatment is now being used successfully. A collagen injection, done as an out-patient procedure, stops the leakage of urine by padding out the tissue of the bladder neck. Pioneered by a urogynecologist at a London hospital, the technique is helpful for women of any age, particularly those who would rather avoid major surgery.

Kegel (pelvic floor) exercises

You can keep the muscles around the vagina, bladder, and anus toned by exercises. Pregnant women are advised to do them before and after the birth. The beauty of the Kegels is that you can do them whenever and wherever you want without anyone knowing. The improvement won't be instantaneous, but after eight weeks of doing them at least three to five times a day you will notice that your control is much better.

YOU REALLY NEED TO KNOW

◆ Women have a short urethra and the opening is close to both the vagina and the anus so this area is prone to infection.

◆ The bladder holds about a pint of urine, but if you get into the habit of emptying it before it is even half full, the muscle tone is affected for the worse.

◆ The pelvic floor is made up of muscles that form a "sling" that supports the bladder, rectum, and uterus. In pregnancy the expanding uterus can put stress on the whole area.

Controlling incontinence

Lifestyle changes

SELF-HELP

✓ One of the easiest ways to manage stress is by taking exercise.

✓ A moderate intake of wine (up to a glass and a half a day) may give some protection against stroke and heart disease and may also protect against Alzheimer's and Parkinson's diseases.

✓ Drink plain water throughout the day to counter your body's normal water loss.

HRT is not a substitute for healthy eating and exercise. While it is healthier at and after menopause to have some body fat (see p. 46), being overweight isn't good for you. The World Health Organization and other health experts are agreed that by changing your eating habits you are likely to reduce your risk of developing heart disease, stroke, diabetes, and some common cancers.

Vitamins and minerals

Vitamins and minerals make the body function at its optimal level. Nutritionists and dieticians say that you should get all you need from a balanced diet but you may not be eating a wide enough variety of foods or they may be altered by disease, processing, or cooking. A diet or lifestyle restricted by illness or age, smoking, or, rarely, taking medicinal drugs that deplete vitamin and mineral levels (HRT is not in this category) can have an effect too.

Should I take supplements?

This depends on your diet. As you get older the antioxidants (vitamins A, C, E, and the mineral selenium) become more important to protect the cells of the body from damage. It is important to heed any warnings that may be given. Vitamin A should not be taken in excess and calcium can leave deposits in the kidneys. Bone-protecting supplements combine calcium with vitamin D, and calcium is formulated with glucosamine and chondroitin (both found naturally in the connective tissue of joints). Usually the body will excrete any calcium it doesn't need—as it will most excess vitamins and minerals—but if you are in any doubt you should ask your doctor or a nutritionist for advice. Supplements give the recommended daily allowance (RDA) on the label.

Move with the times

Inactivity will eventually lead to immobility. The best type of exercise will build strength and stamina, increase flexibility, and help your balance and concentration.

Improving bone density and muscle strength should be a priority at and after menopause. The exercises, sports, and activities that do this best are tennis, badminton, brisk walking, jogging, climbing stairs, step aerobics, trampolining, and line dancing. Swimming and cycling, though good for overall fitness, are not weight-bearing. You should aim to breathe deeply and move well, both of which will lift your spirits since they increase your levels of serotonin (a brain hormone that affects mood).

TAKE REGULAR EXERCISE

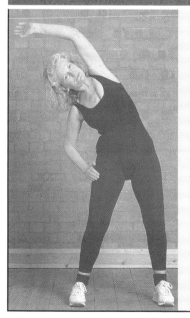

During menopause and after, exercise should be a regular activity—30 minutes a day, or at least three times a week, is recommended to keep you physically fit. Some simple rules are: walk instead of drive, climb stairs instead of taking the elevator, and play a sport instead of watching it on TV.

YOU REALLY NEED TO KNOW

◆ Apart from improved diet and increased exercise, managing stress, stopping smoking, and avoiding excess alcohol are considered the three most important contributions you can make to your own wellbeing.

◆ Drinking excess alcohol is linked to a variety of illnesses, including those of the stomach, liver, kidneys, breasts, bladder, and bowel. "Safe" limits for a woman are one to one and a half drinks a day or less.

Understanding the jargon

Many of the terms that you will meet when finding out more about HRT and menopause may be unfamiliar to you. This page gives definitions of the words you are most likely to come across.

AMENORRHEA—absence of periods

CERVIX—the neck of the womb (uterus)

CLIMACTERIC—the time during which menstruation is irregular and eventually ceases

CORTICOSTEROIDS—powerful steroid drugs that are used to reduce inflammation in the body

D&C—(dilatation and curettage) surgical procedure to scrape out or check the womb lining

DYSPAREUNIA—painful intercourse

ENDOMETRIOSIS—abnormal growth of the womb lining (endometrium) outside the womb

FIBROIDS—benign growth in the womb

FOLLICLE—sac for eggs in the ovary

FSH—follicle-stimulating hormone produced by the pituitary to stimulate the ovary to produce eggs

GONADS—female (and male) sex glands

HYSTERECTOMY—surgical removal of the womb

ISOFLAVONES—weak estrogen-like chemicals

LH—luteinizing hormone from the pituitary, which stimulates the ovary to produce progesterone

MAMMOGRAPHY—procedure in which the breasts are X rayed to screen for abnormal changes

MENARCHE—start of menstruation (periods)

MENORRHAGIA—heavy periods

OOPHORECTOMY—surgical removal of an ovary

OVARY—female sex gland

PERIMENOPAUSE—the time around menopause

POLYP—growth, usually benign, in the womb lining or at the cervix

PROLAPSE—downward slippage (most commonly of the womb, neck of the bladder, or lower bowel)

SPECULUM—instrument used to open the vagina for an internal examination or Pap smear

URETHRA—tube that carries urine from the bladder out of the body

UTERUS—the womb, a muscular organ under the influence of the reproductive hormones

VAGINISMUS—involuntary paralysis of the vaginal area, which prevents sex or internal examination

VULVA—describes the area around the vagina

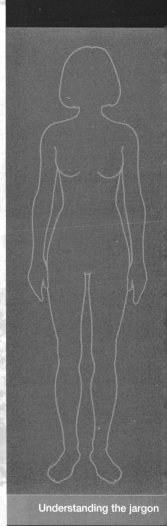

Understanding the jargon

Useful addresses

NATIONAL OSTEOPOROSIS FOUNDATION
1150 17th Street, NW
Washington, DC 20036
Call: (800) 223-9994 or
(202) 223-2226
Publication on osteoporosis.
Contacts for local support groups.

OLDER WOMEN'S LEAGUE
666 11th St, NW, Suite 700
Washington, DC 20001
Call: (202) 783-6686 or
(800) TAKE-OWL
Publish status report on
osteoporosis, fact sheets, and a
resource guide.

ADMINISTRATION ON AGING
330 Independence Avenue, SW
Washington, DC 20201
Call: (202) 619-0641

NATIONAL INSTITUTION ON AGING INFORMATION CENTER
PO Box 8057
Gaitnersburg, MD 20898-8057
Call: (800) 222-2225
Publishes *Resource Directory for Older People* and *Who? What? Where?* resources for Women's Health and Aging, and *Age Pages*.

NATIONAL WOMEN'S HEALTH NETWORK
514 10th St NW, Suite 402
Washington, DC 20004
Call: (202) 347-1140
Educational organization.

NATIONAL ASSOCIATION FOR CONTINENCE
Call: (800) BLADDER
Web site: http://www.nafc.org

Index

Index

Acknowledgments
Photographs: Science Photo Library: 12, 29, 30, 32, 42, 44, 68-69;
Tony Stone Images: 26-27, 37, 70-71. All other photographs: George Taylor.
Models: Patricia Monahan, Wendy Dear. Illustrations: Coral Mula.
Information about Raloxifene p. 59 Brigham and Women's Hospital, Boston, Mass.